1 CHERRIES

is very rich in vitamins C, A and fiber. Consistent intake of Vitamin C can help reduce uric acid levels by up to 50 percent, and control inflammation of gout-ravaged joints, which is a primary cause of severe gout pain.

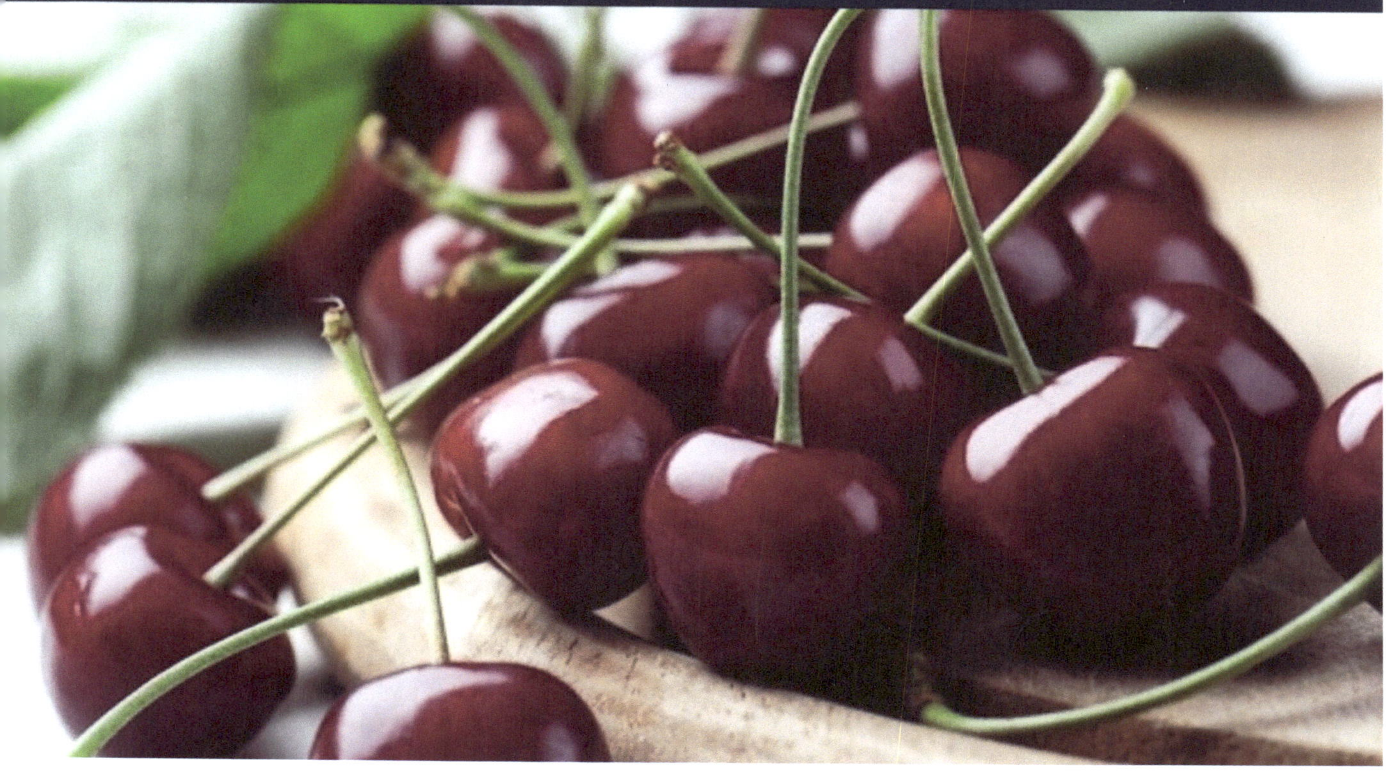

2
AVOCADO

have more potassium per 100 grams than bananas. This is very important for gout sufferers since potassium helps excrete uric acid from the body. This will also help gout sufferers avoid high blood pressure which puts them at an increased risk of heart attack, stroke and kidney failure.

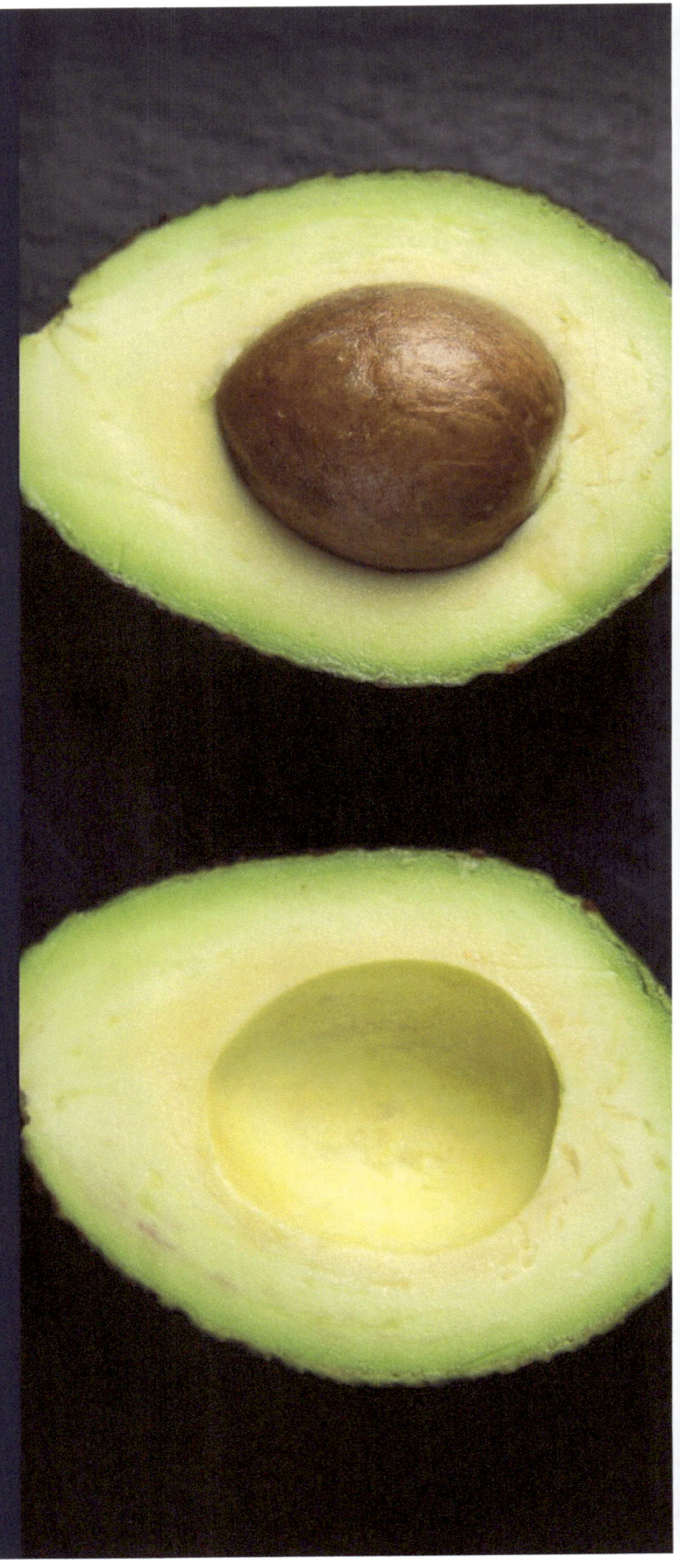

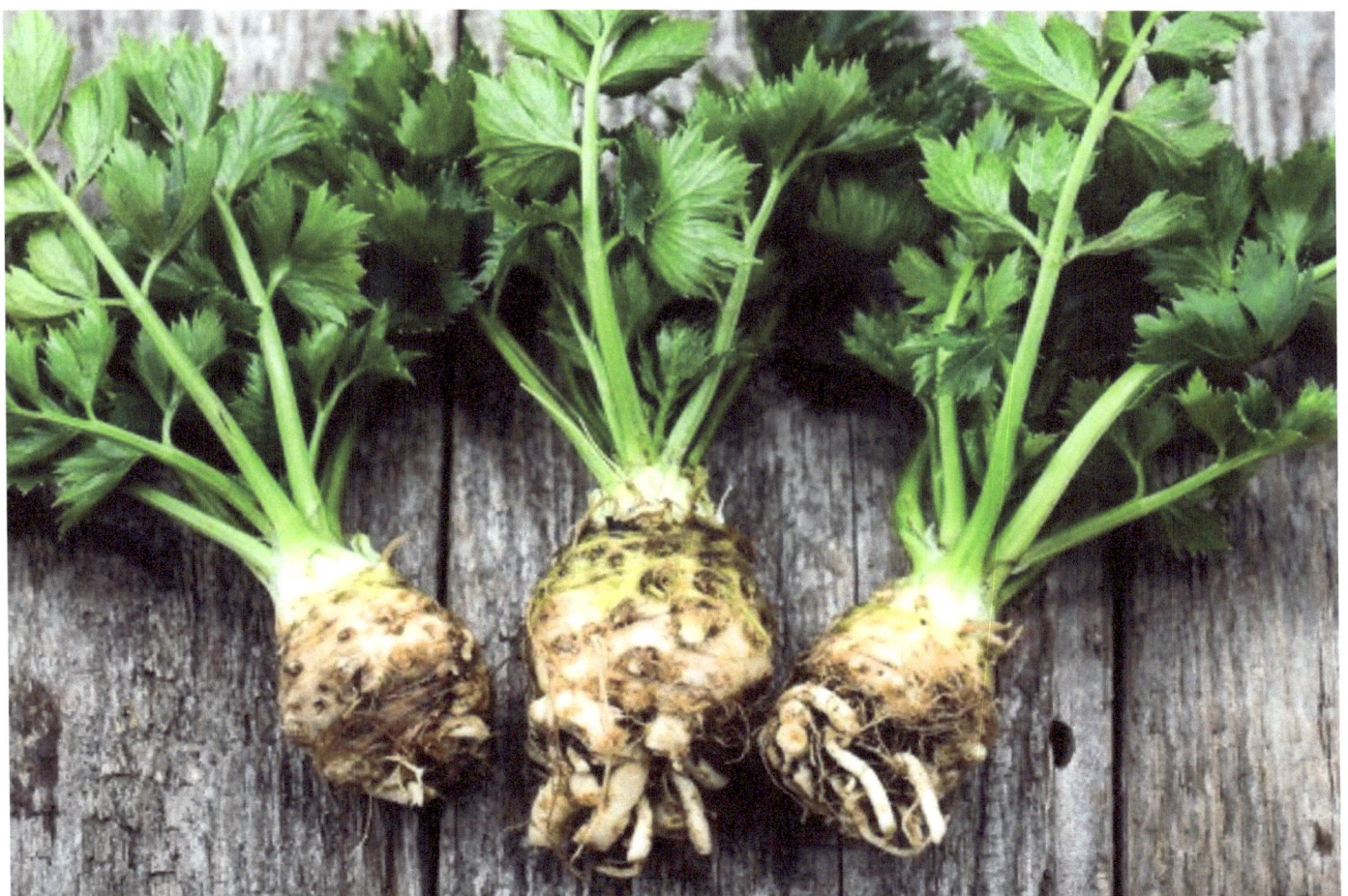

3
CELERY
IS THE PERFECT GOUT-FIGHTING FOOD, BECAUSE IT:

1. Acts as an anti-inflammatory, helping stop the pain of gout attacks.

2. Is a diuretic, promoting the excretion of uric acid through urine.

3. Helps manage uric acid by acting as an xanthine oxidase (XO) inhibitor, similar to allopurinol.

4. Is highly alkalizing, which helps reduce uric acid buildup.

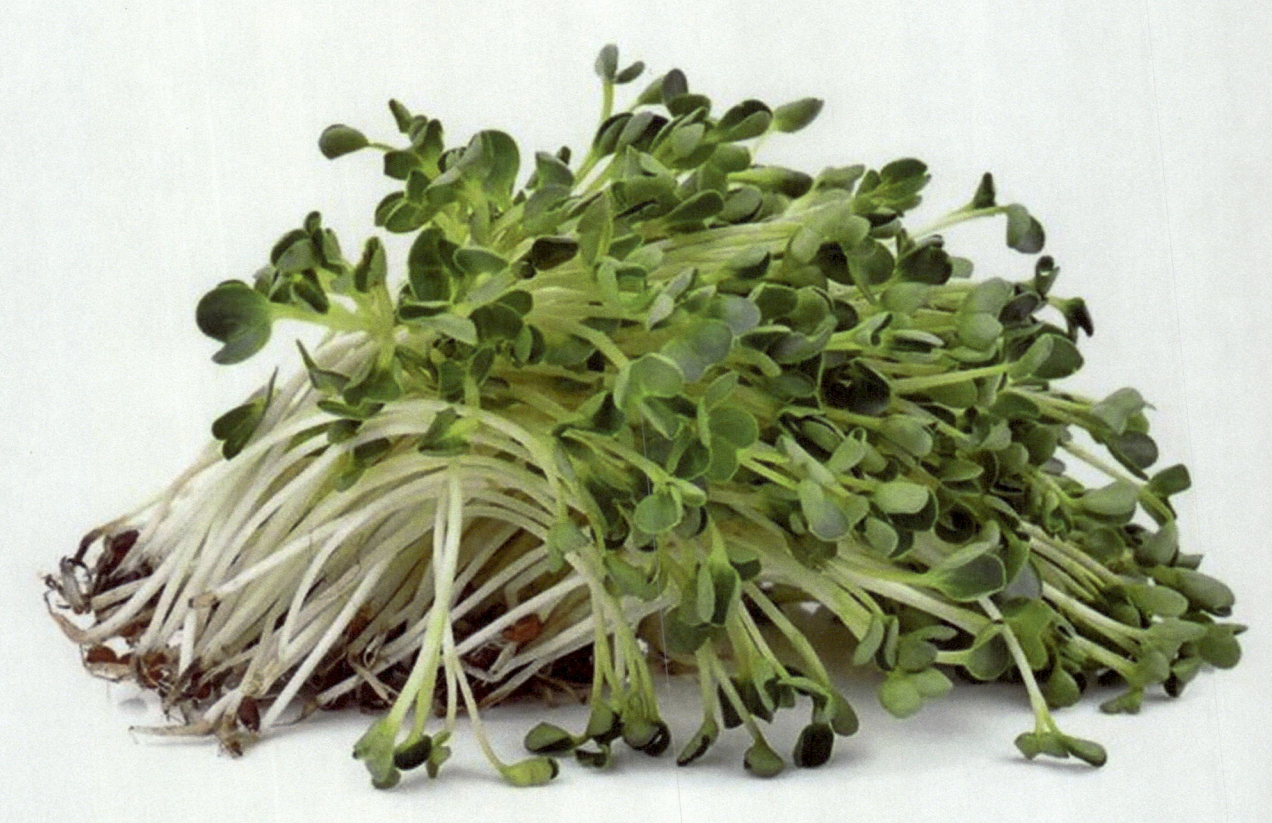

4
ALFALFA

the leaves of the alfalfa plant are rich in minerals, essential amino acids and nutrients (phosphorous, calcium, magnesium, potassium, and carotene which actively promote kidney function) and other minerals. All these minerals are diuretic in nature and, therefore help to remove fluid accumulations in muscle tissue and joints. Alfalfa is an excellent natural source of most vitamins: A, B1, B6, B8, B12, C, D, E, K1, P, and U. Alfalfa is also higher in protein than any other plant food. Alfalfa works by helping to neutralize and reduce high uric acid levels in your blood, but it also has natural anti-inflammatory and antioxidant properties, making it a good choice to consume alfalfa for the gout sufferer. What alfalfa does very well is increase uric acid levels in your urine which can help reduce the excess amount of uric acid available to crystallize and give you a gout attack

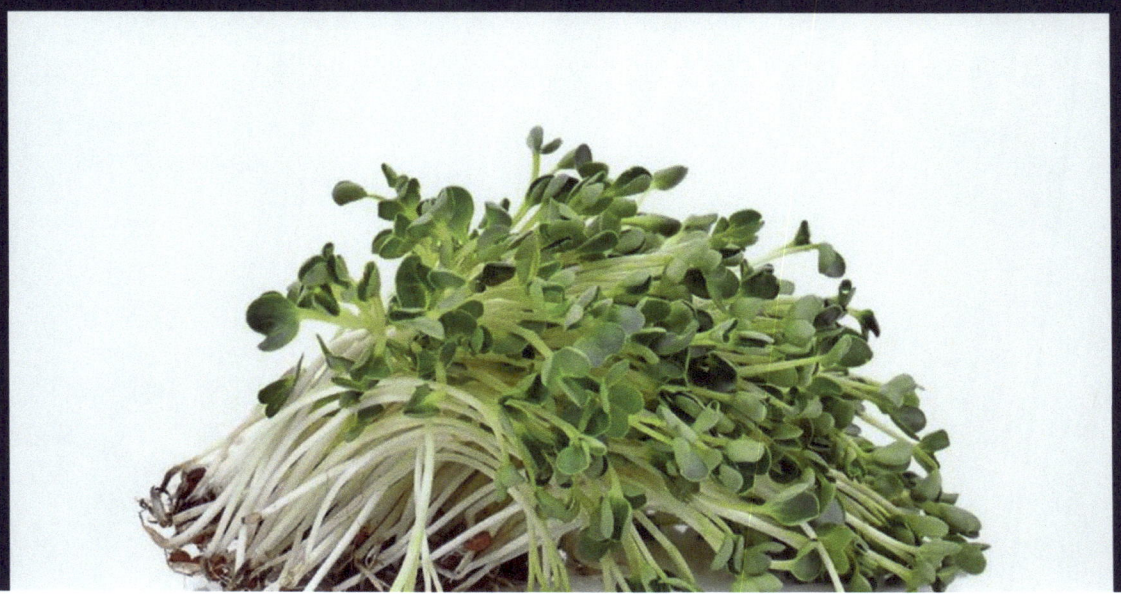

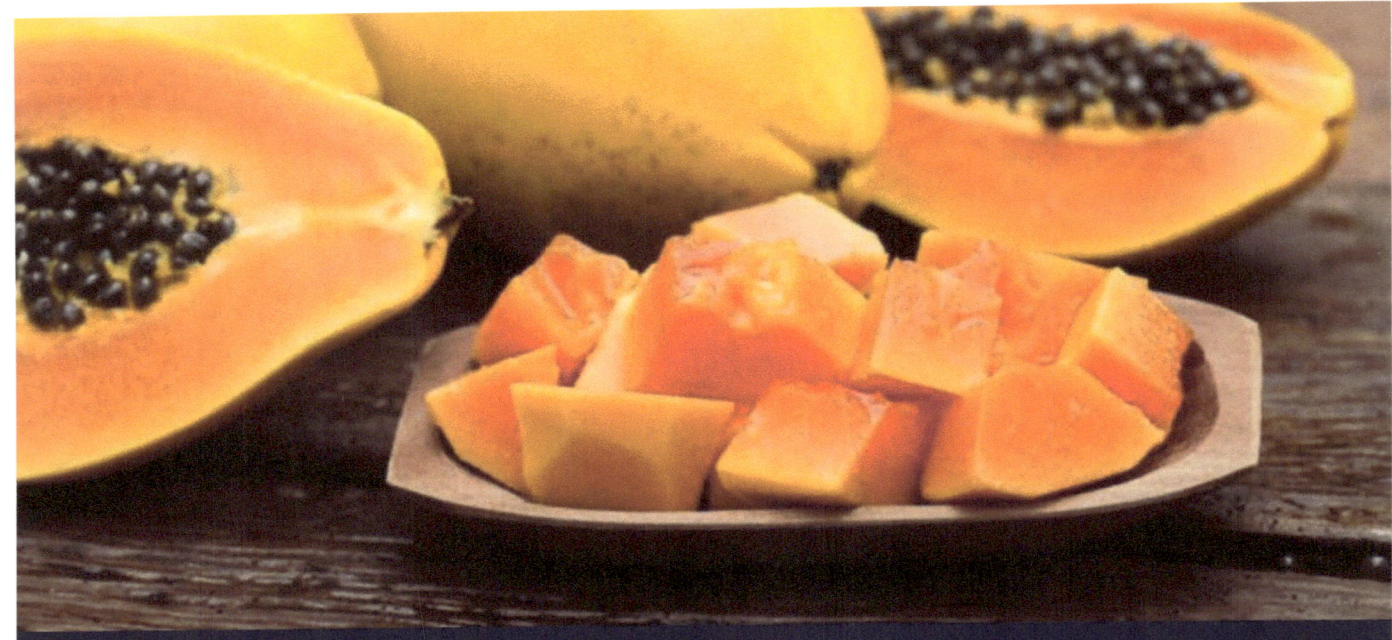

5 PAPAYA

is very good for us gout sufferers since it contains "papain" a proteolytic enzyme which is a natural anti-inflammatory, helping keep the body in an alkaline state, preventing the buildup of uric acid in the blood. Basically, papaya helps you digest proteins from meat, poultry, fish and other foods. Since papaya is rich in vitamin C, it is a beneficial food for the gout sufferer. Another key health benefit for gout sufferers is that papaya is also very high in vitamin C. Papaya is also rich in antioxidant nutrients such as carotenes, flavonoids; the B vitamins, folate and pantothenic acid. In minerals, it contains potassium, copper, and magnesium and fiber.

6
PINEAPPLE

has a sturdy stem and it contains bromelain which is an enzyme or better yet a mix of a number of different protein digesting enzymes. Pineapple is also loaded with vitamin C, a strong antioxidant. Bromelain causes the uric acid crystals to decompose thus relieving you from the pain associated with gout. If taken regularly, bromelain may also prevent repeated gout attacks.

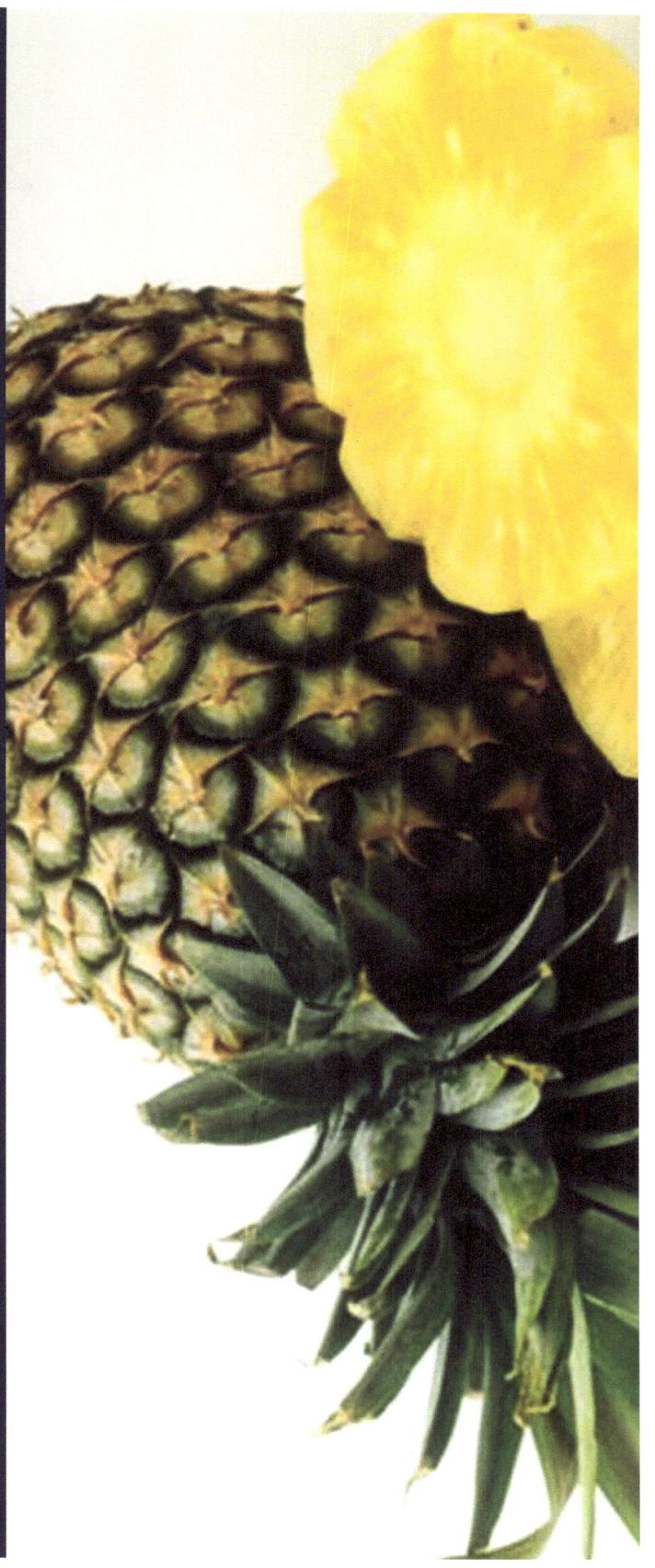

7 POMEGRANATE

the most important health benefit of pomegranate though is it's powerful antioxidant properties which help reduce uric acid in the blood. Another important fact about pomegranates is that their content carries acids like citric and malic acid. Citric acid helps eliminate uric acid and its salts through the urine helping gout sufferers.

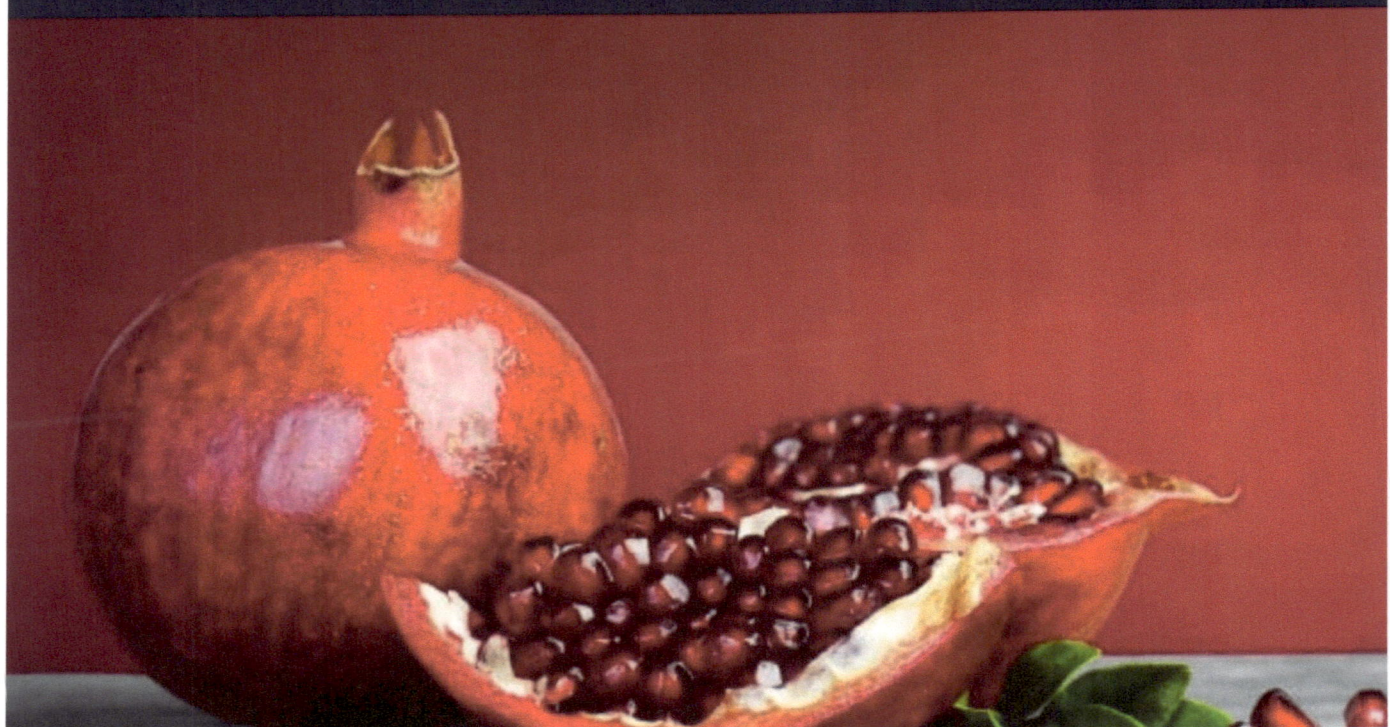

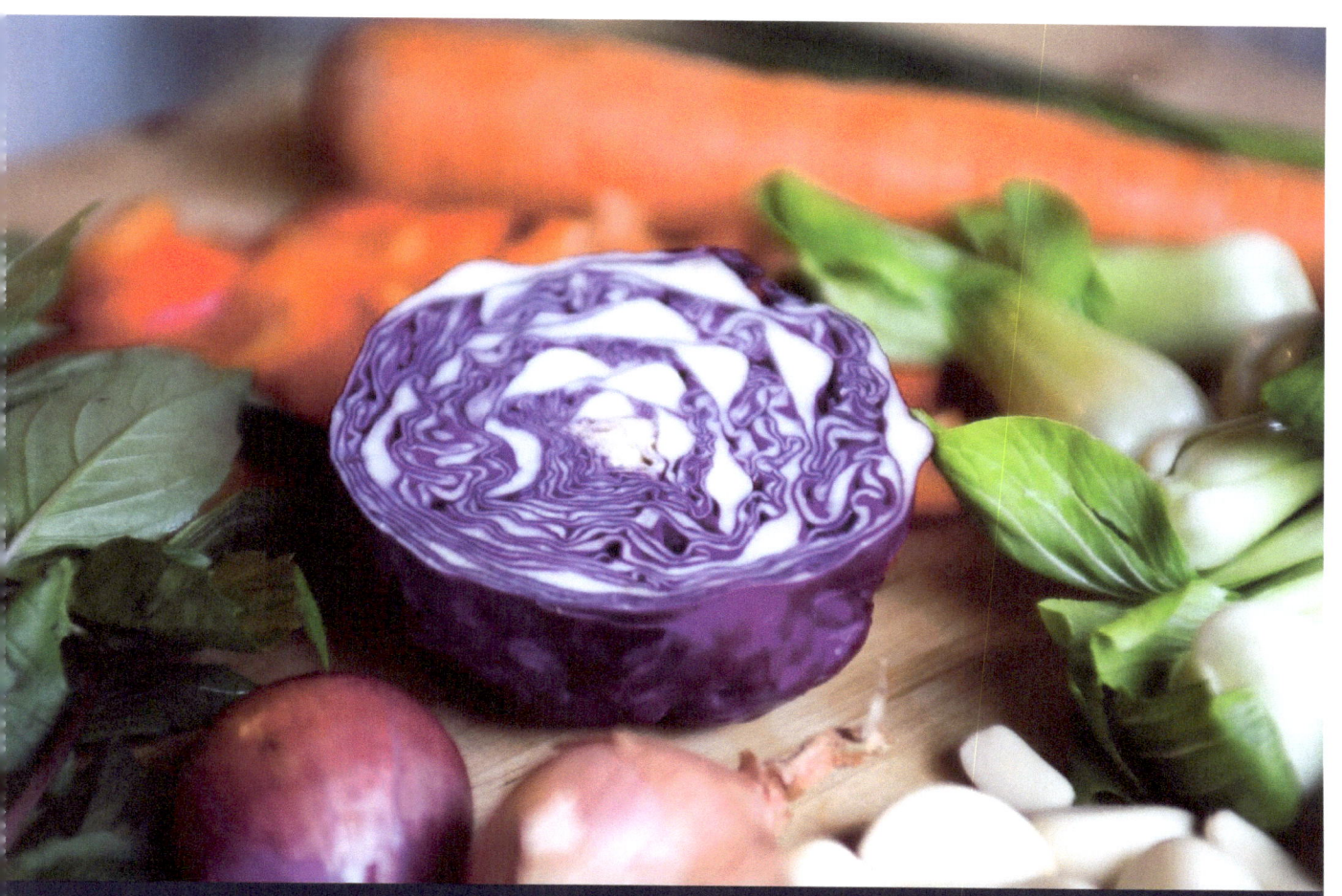

CABBAGE

is high in vitamins K, C, B6 and is loaded with minerals like potassium, manganese and iron. Cabbage is also known to purify the blood and removes toxins helping lower uric acid levels in your blood. In addition, the anthocyanins that are found in red cabbage have strong anti-inflammatory compounds. An enzyme that is in the cabbage leaves helps get rid of the crystals that are nestled around the joint.

8

9 BASIL

is also considered as a medicinal herb since it is high in vitamins K, A and vitamin C, manganese, copper, iron and calcium. Basil is known to stimulate our kidneys and helps lower uric acid levels in your blood helping gout and arthritis sufferers. It is effective in blocking the signals that lead to inflammation associated with gout and arthritis.

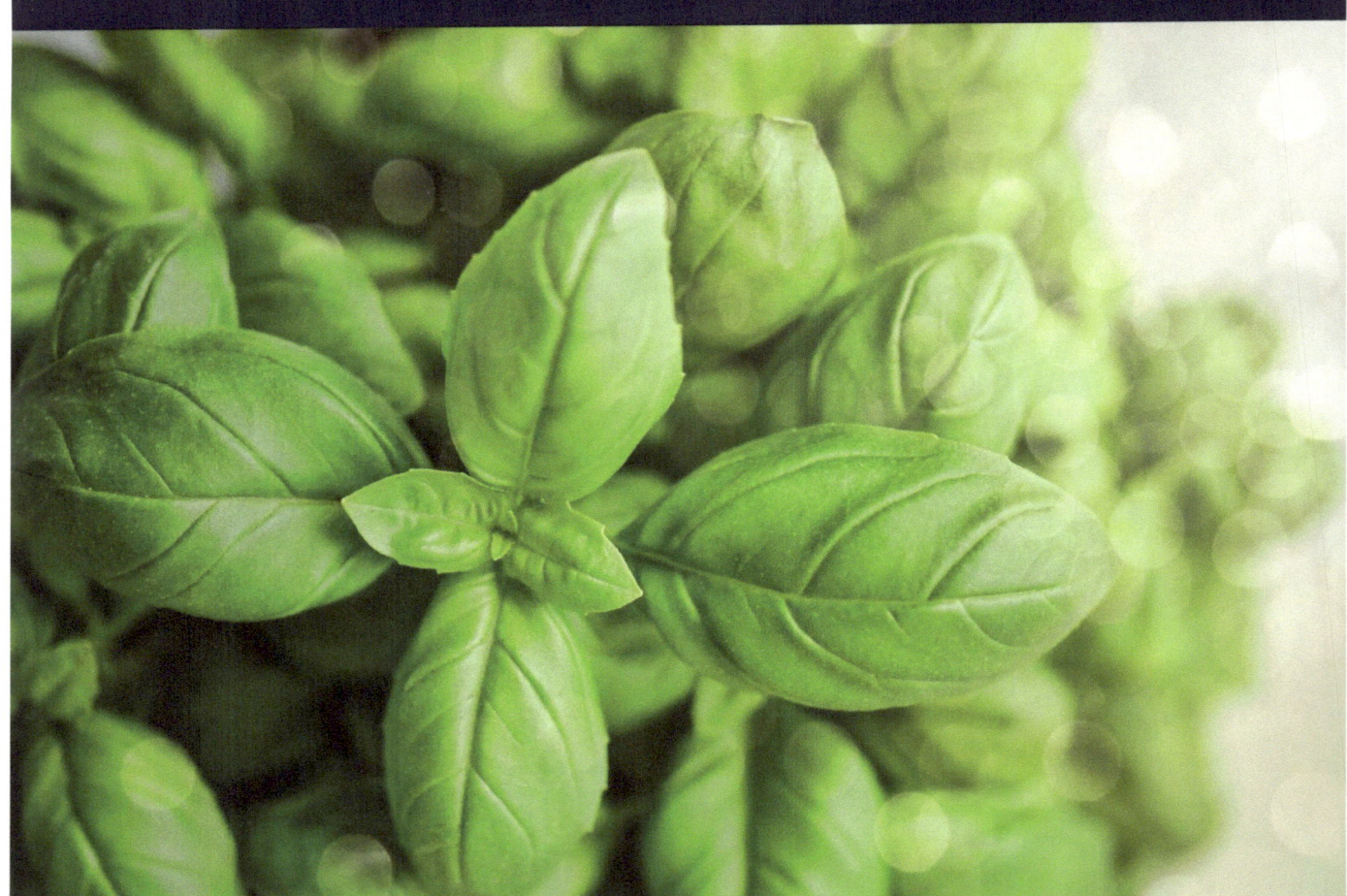

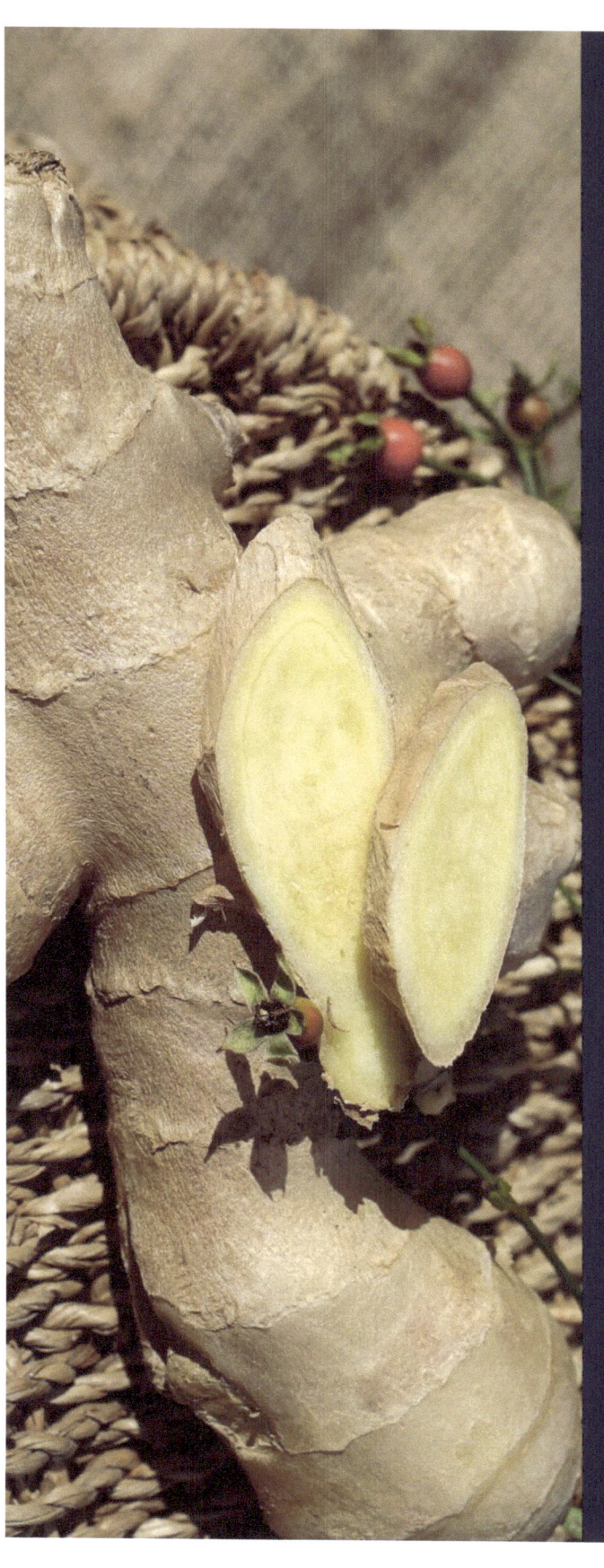

10
GINGER

though packs full of health benefits especially relieving oneself from gastrointestinal symptoms, motion sickness, and seasickness reducing the symptoms of nausea, dizziness and vomiting. Ginger's strong anti-inflammatory compounds, help patients with gout.

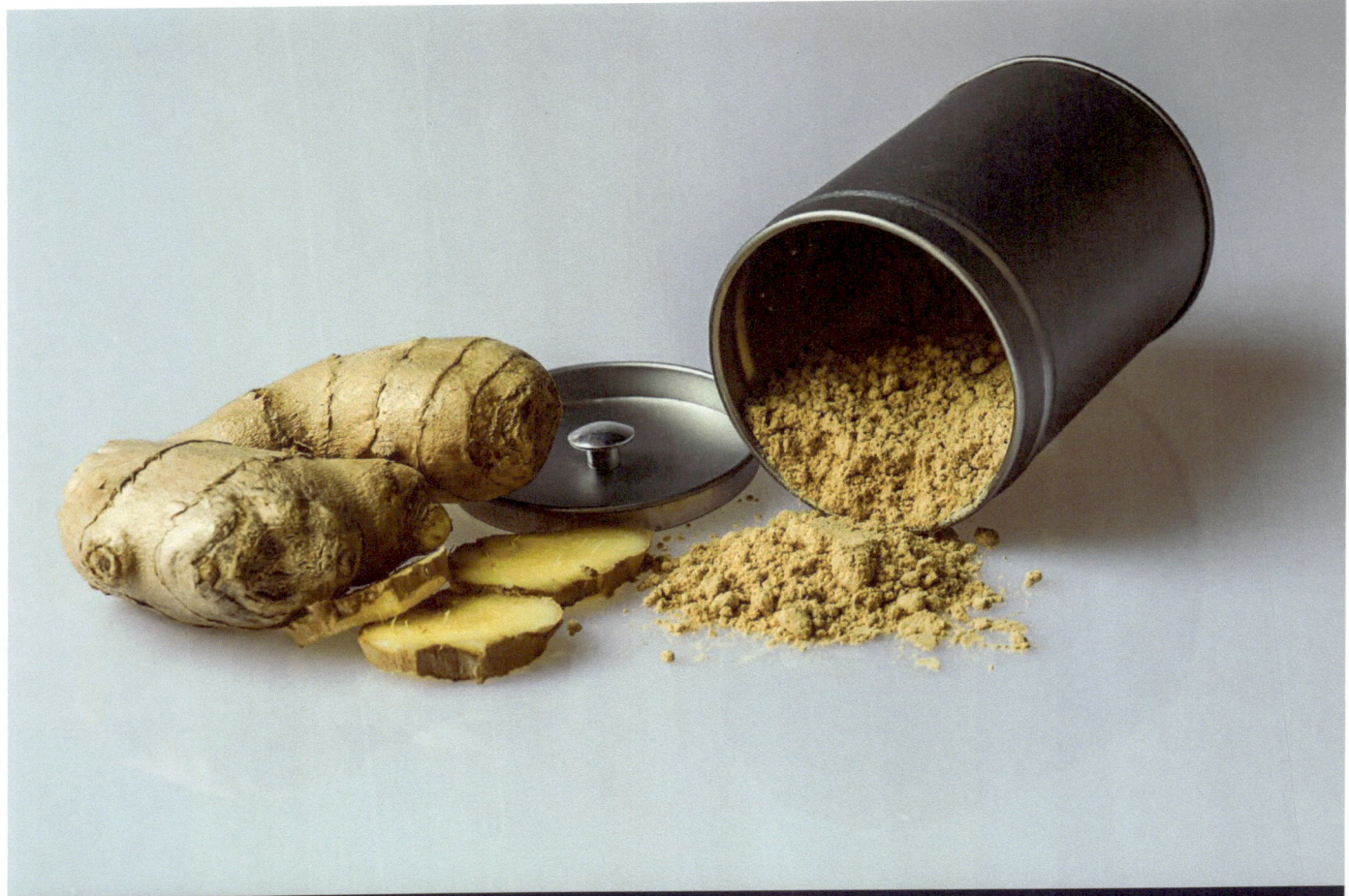

TURMERIC

11

though packs full of health benefits especially relieving oneself from gastrointestinal symptoms, motion sickness, and seasickness reducing the symptoms of nausea, dizziness and vomiting. Ginger's strong anti-inflammatory compounds, help patients with gout.

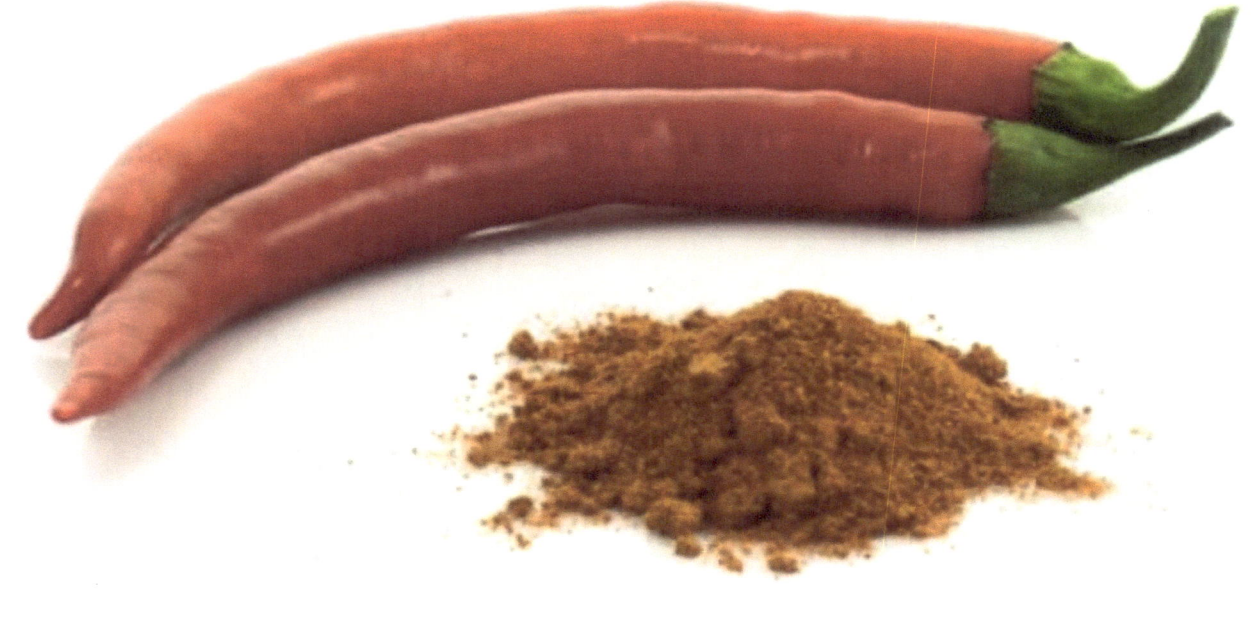

12
CAYENNE PEPPER

can be used to treat many ailments like heartburn, fever, flatulence (helping stimulate the digestive tract) nausea, tonsillitis, migraines, colds and the flu (helping break up and move congested mucus), supports weight loss, is considered a anti-cancer agent, helps blood circulation and prevents factors leading to the formation of blood clots helping reduce the risk of heart attack or stroke which many gout sufferers are at risk of.

13
TOMATOES

contain a rich source of antioxidants, is high in vitamin C and a lot of water, but water is important for us gout sufferers. Tomatoes are a low purine food, sugar and carbs as well.

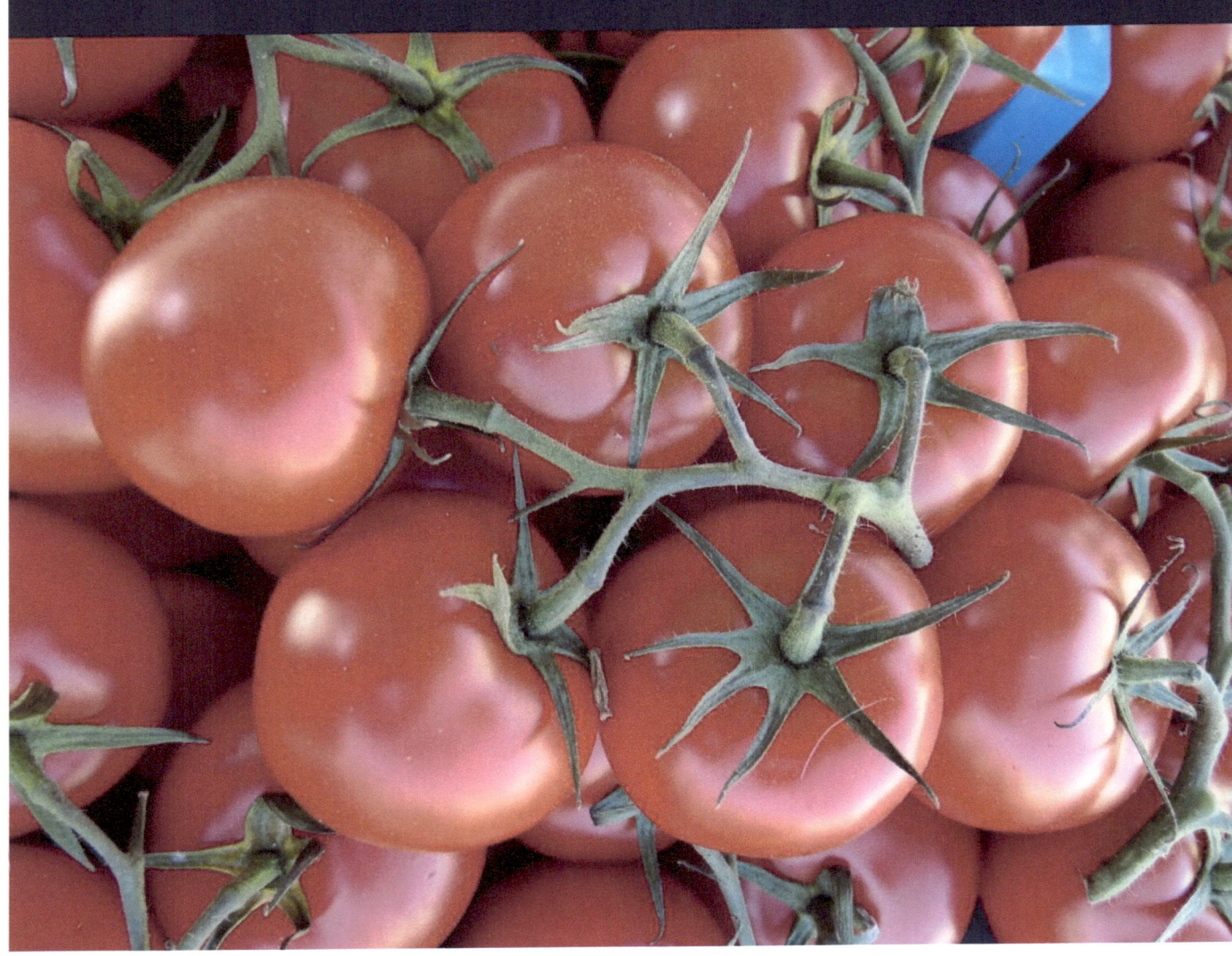

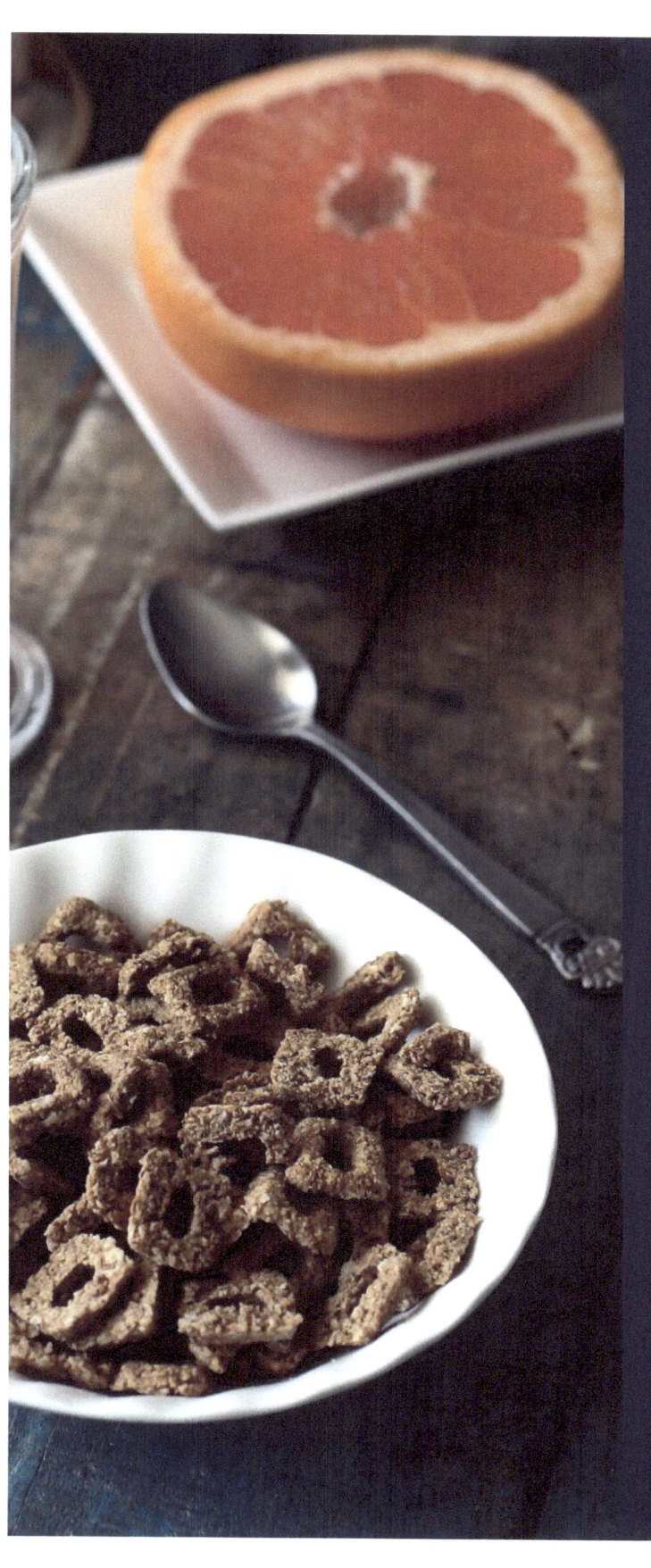

14 FIBER

helps people suffering from gout. It helps keep normal bowel movements and maintain good bowel health. It helps lower cholesterol in the blood by promoting the good cholesterol (HDL) over the bad (LDL). A high fiber diet helps control your blood sugar levels decreasing your risk of developing diabetes later in life and helps you maintain your ideal weight which is very healthy.

15 APPLES

are extremely rich in antioxidants, flavanoids and dietary fiber. Appeles are a low purine, also are high in vitamin C which has been shown to lower uric acid levels. Apples can combat against inflammatory diseases. Is best to stick with Granny Smith apples since it also has the lowest sugar content from all variety of apples.

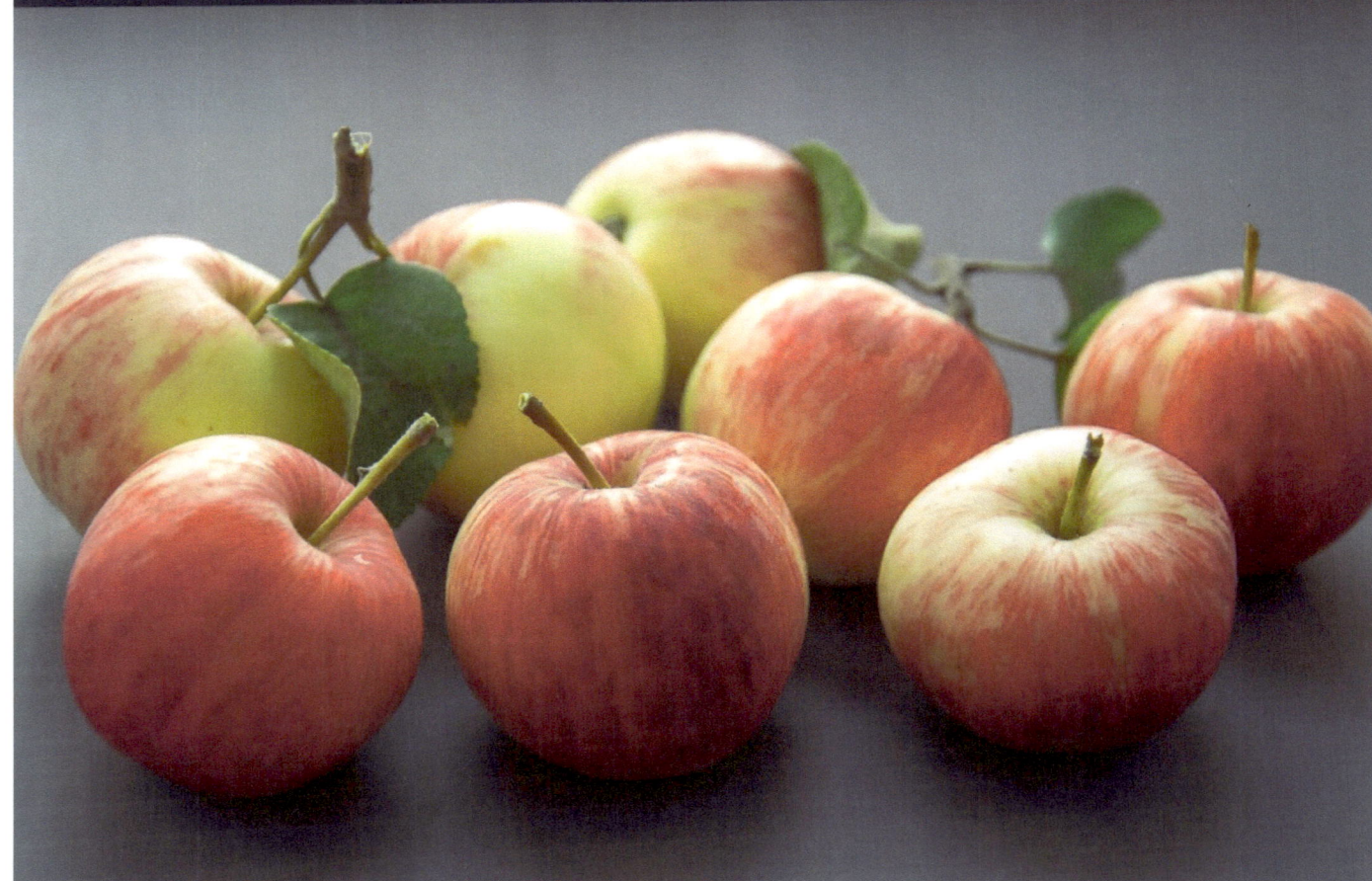

16
BERRIES

are naturally low in purines. The ascorbic acid in berries is very effective in repairing cell damage caused by gout. All berries are high in flavonoids which possess strong anti-inflammatory and antioxidant properties. The Vitamin C in berries is good for gout sufferers and it being effective in reducing uric acid in the body in order to prevent urate crystals. Blueberries like all berries are high in antioxidants which fights inflammation in the body and are important because they neutralize the free radicals that damage your tissues usually in the big toe.

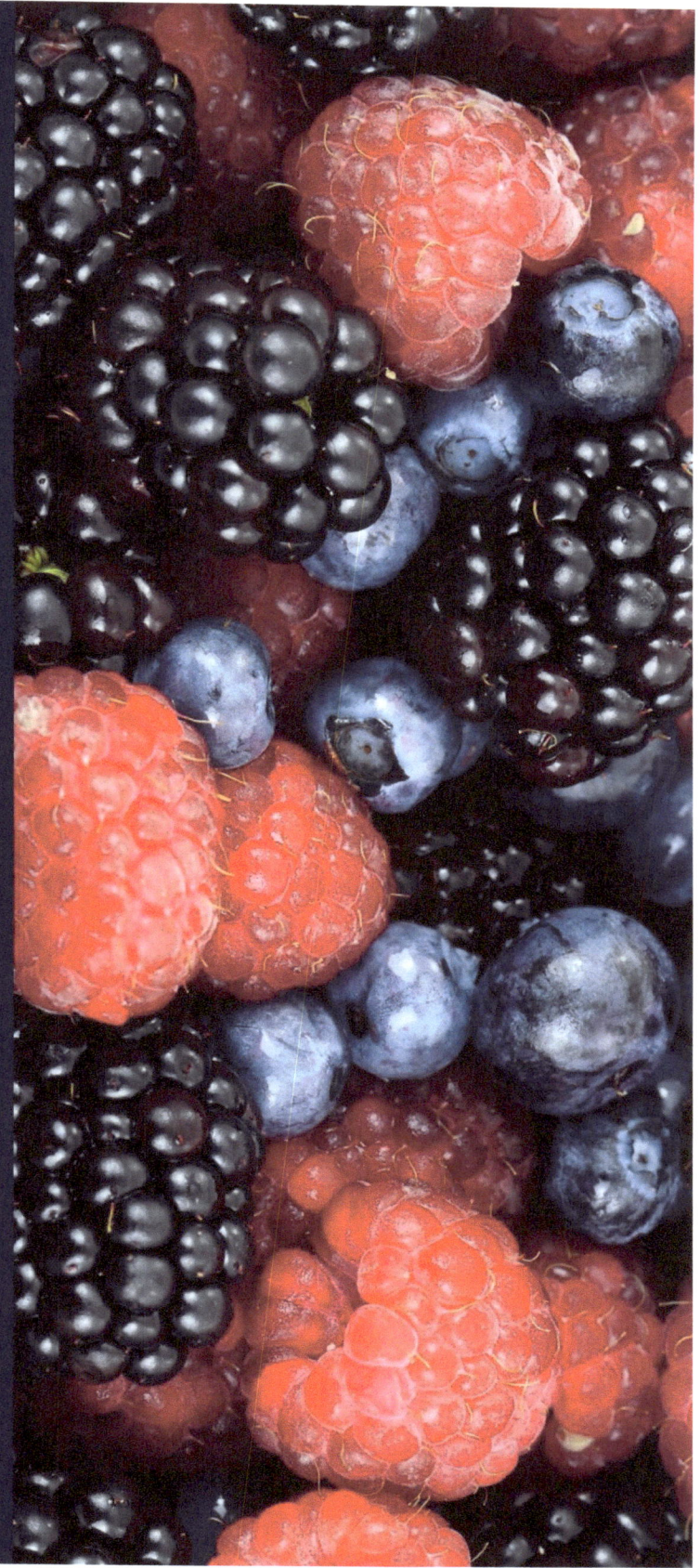

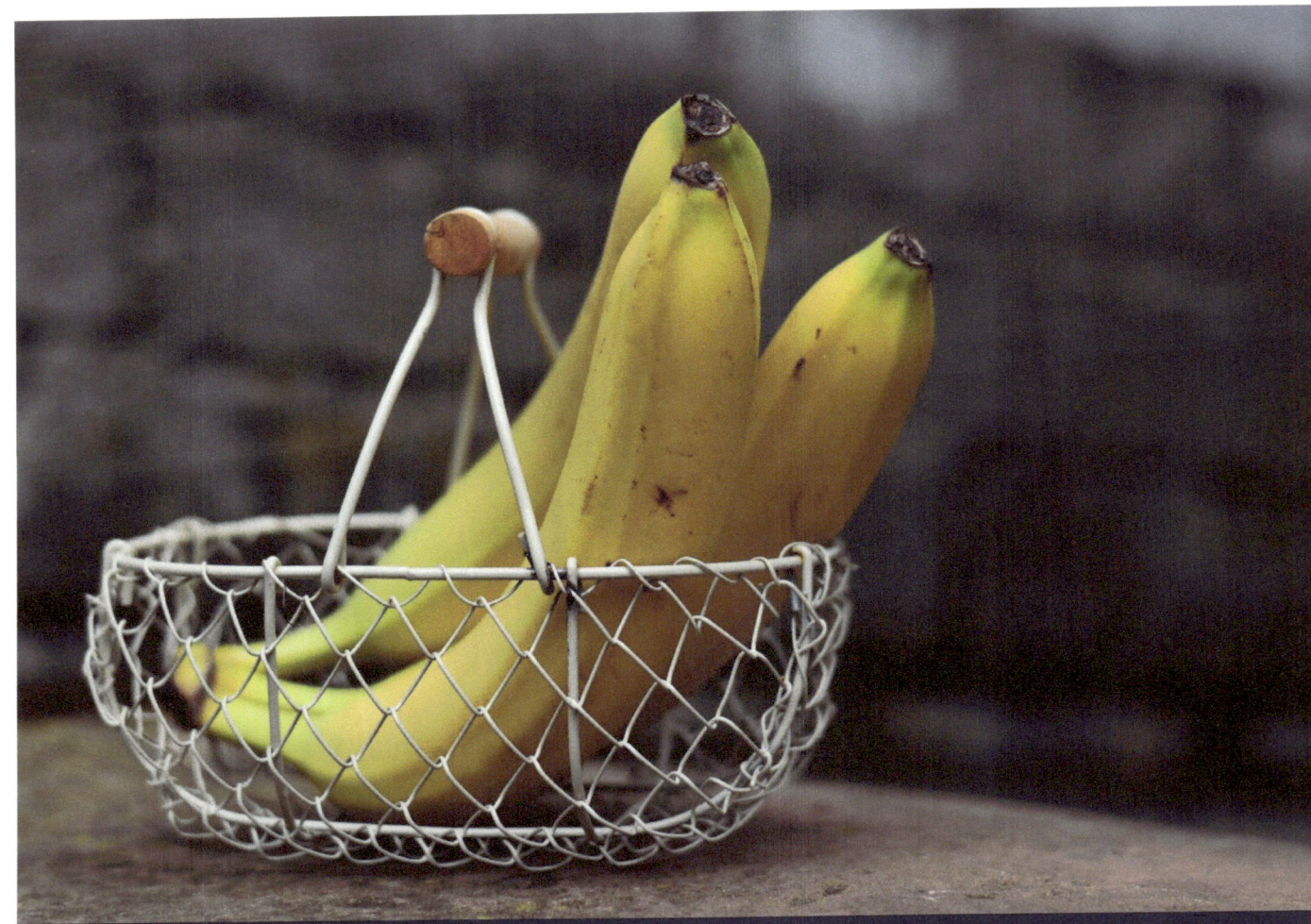

BANANAS

17

one banana has about 105 calories and is low on sugar but very high in vitamins B6, vitamin C, fiber, magnesium, folic acid and potassium; which is very beneficial to the gout sufferer and should be part of your daily diet. Bananas assist in converting uric acid into liquid form which can then be filtered by the kidneys and excreted through your urine avoiding the crystallization in your joints causing gout symptoms.

18 NUTS

the oils in nuts are very high in healthy fats helping reduce inflammation and pain in the body from gout having. Many nuts are also very rich in omega-3 fatty acids, vitamin E which stops the development of plaques in your arteries

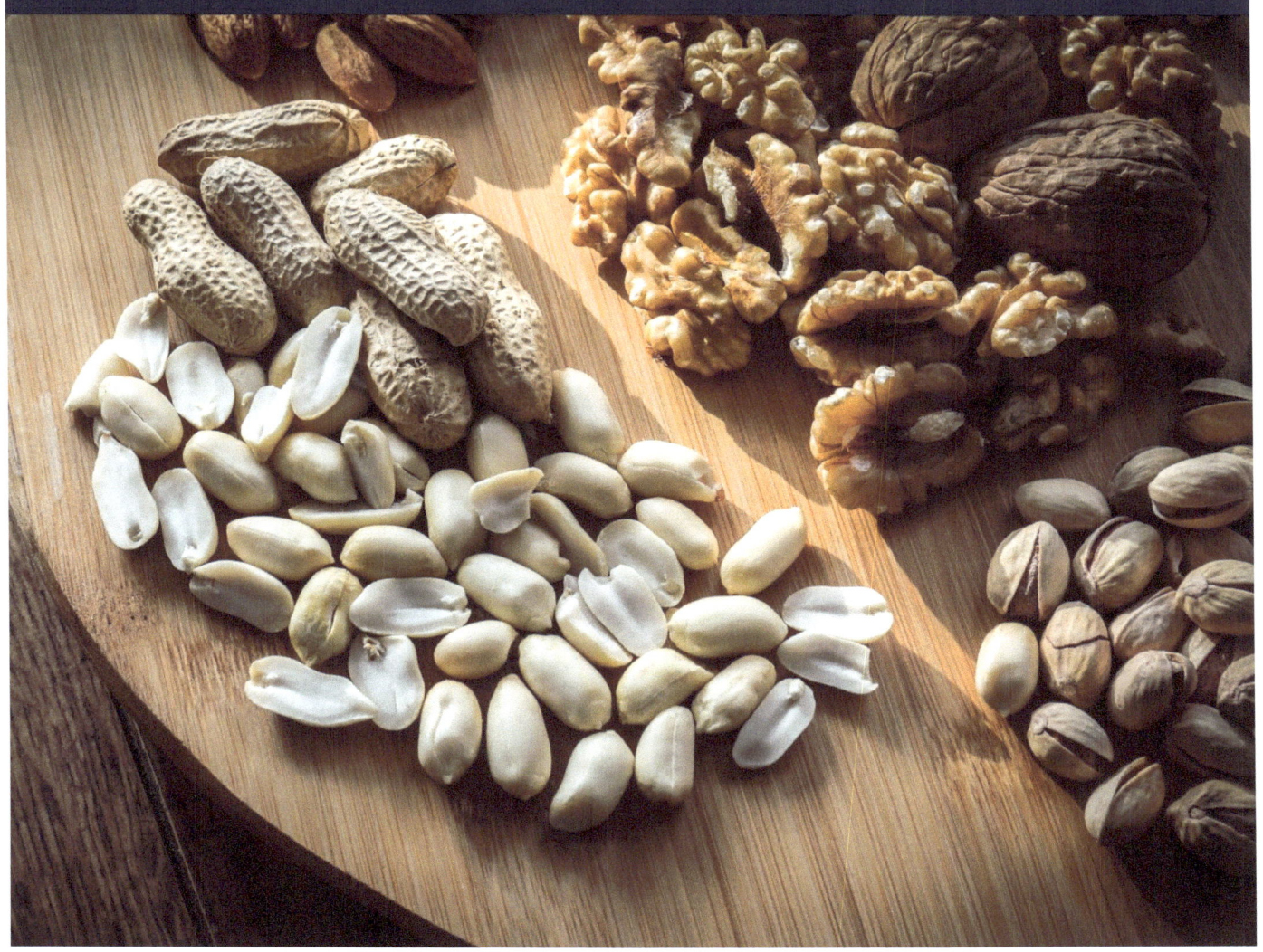

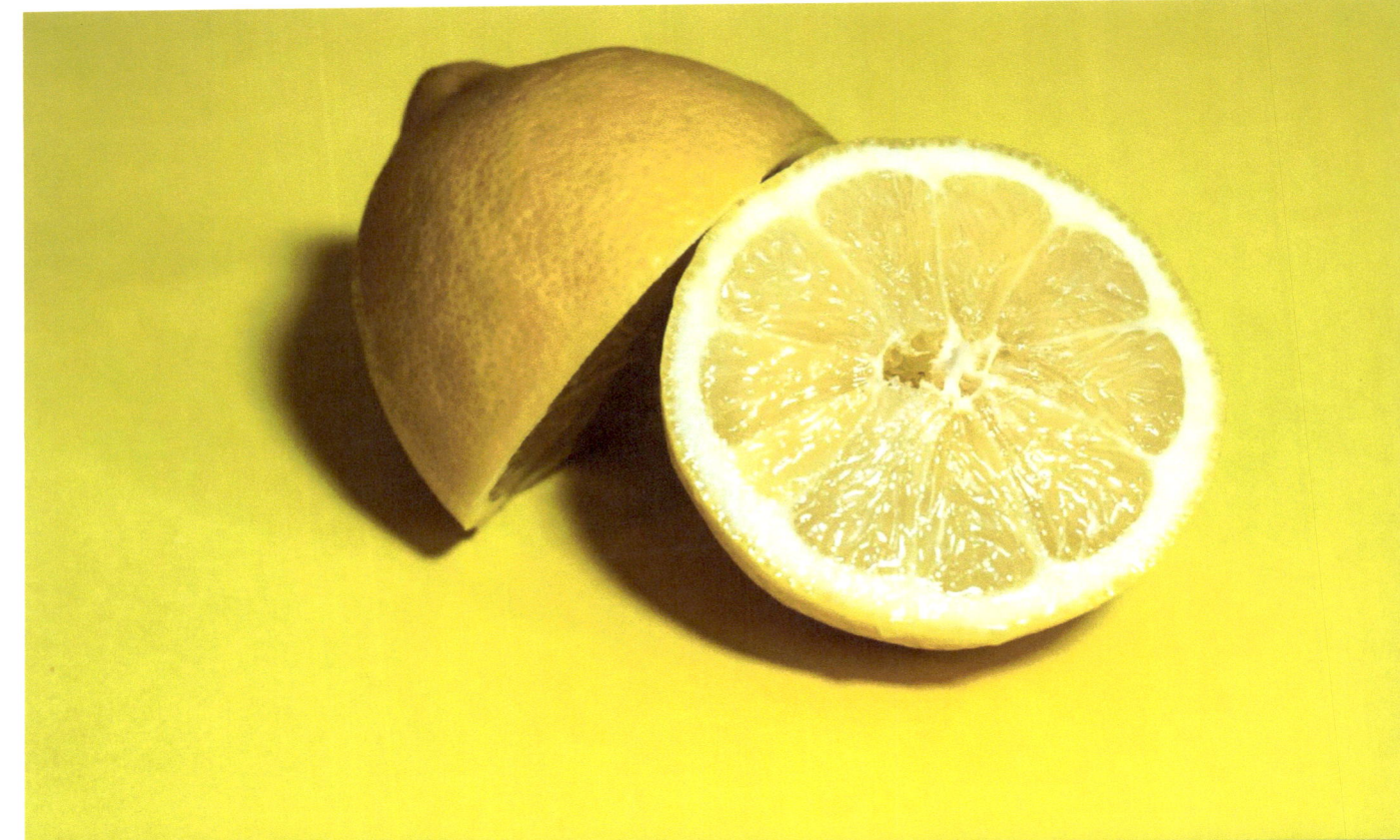

LEMON

19
is naturally high in vitamin C which is a well known natural remedy for gout and also has some vitamin B complex. Help to dissolve uric acid in your blood due to the higher levels of citric acid providing you with relief from a gout attack. One way to improve the body's acidity and remove it is by alkalinizing the urine and lemon juice stimulates the formation of calcium carbonate, which neutralizes acids like uric acid.

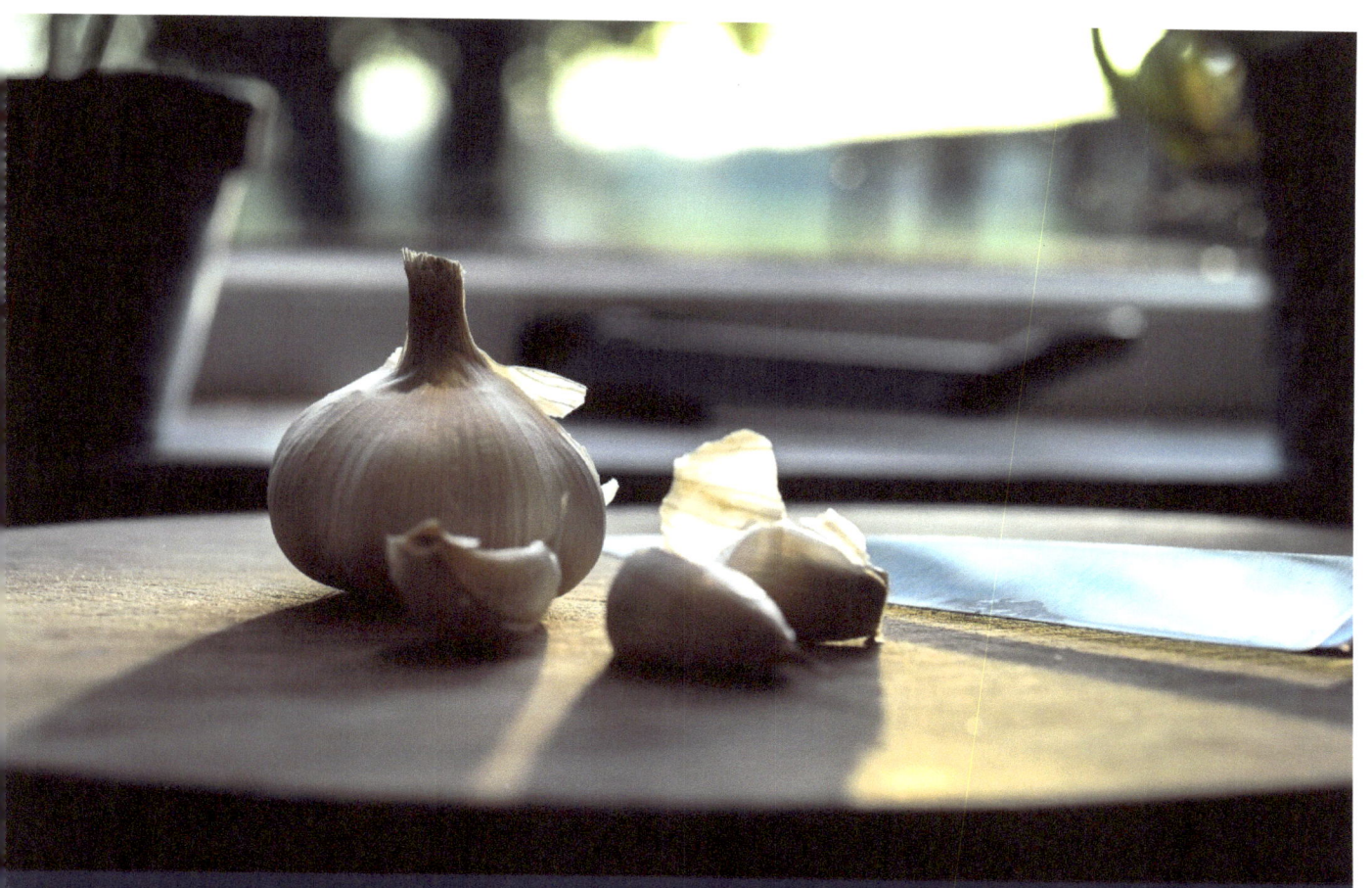

GARLIC

20

has anti-inflammatory action, antioxidant property. This property for garlic can prevent oxidative damage caused by free radicals in joints affected by gout. It is a natural anti-microbial agent and protects joints. Garlic can be used for the treatment of gout as it contains sulphur compounds that show efficient anti-inflammatory activity.

21
CARROT

is an excellent source of pro-vitamin A, vitamins C, D, E, K, B1 and B6. It is rich with biotin, potassium, calcium, magnesium, phosphorus, organic sodium and some trace minerals. It is alkalizing and supports kidney health. The healing properties in carrot juices are helpful for cleansing and filtering the kidneys which neutralizes uric acid.

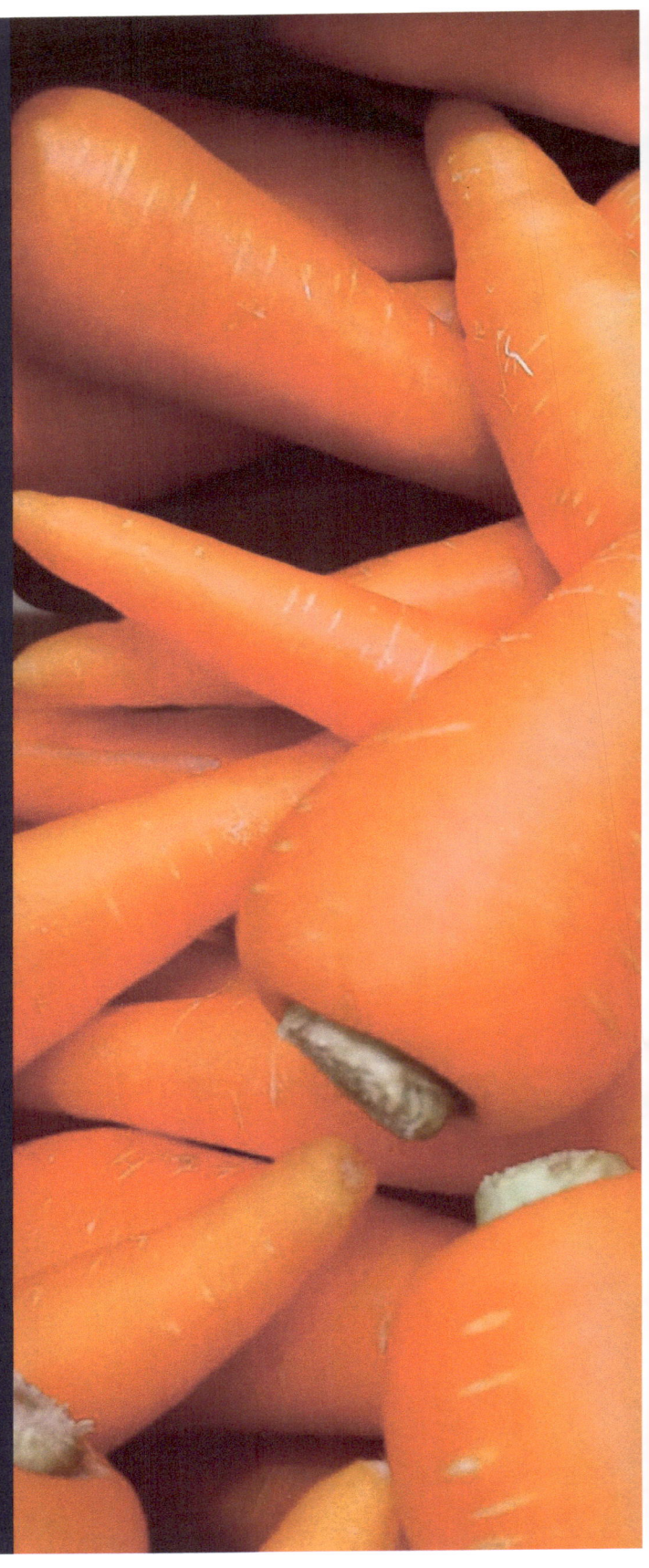

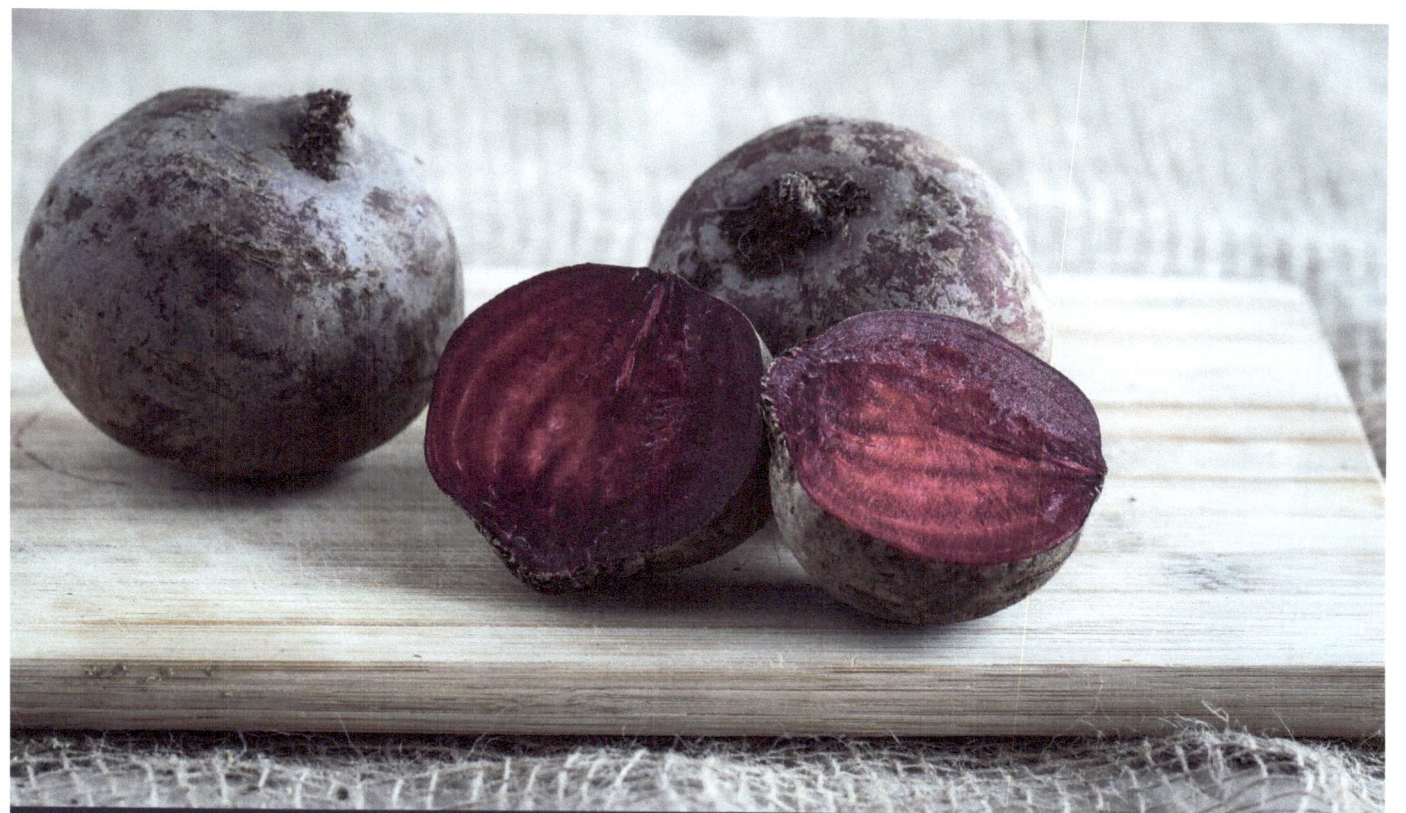

22 BEET

are very powerful cleansers and builders of the blood. Beets are loaded with vitamins A, B1, B2, B6 and C. The greens have a higher content of iron compared to spinach. They are also an excellent source of calcium, magnesium, copper, phosphorus, sodium and iron. Beet helps eliminate uric acid and its salts through the urine helping gout sufferers.

23 SEEDS

are an excellent source of protein in a gout diet, because:

Most seeds are low in purine content.

The oils in seeds are high in healthy fats, which helps reduce the inflammation and pain of gout.

Seeds are good sources of the vitamins and minerals needed to make your body gout-proof.

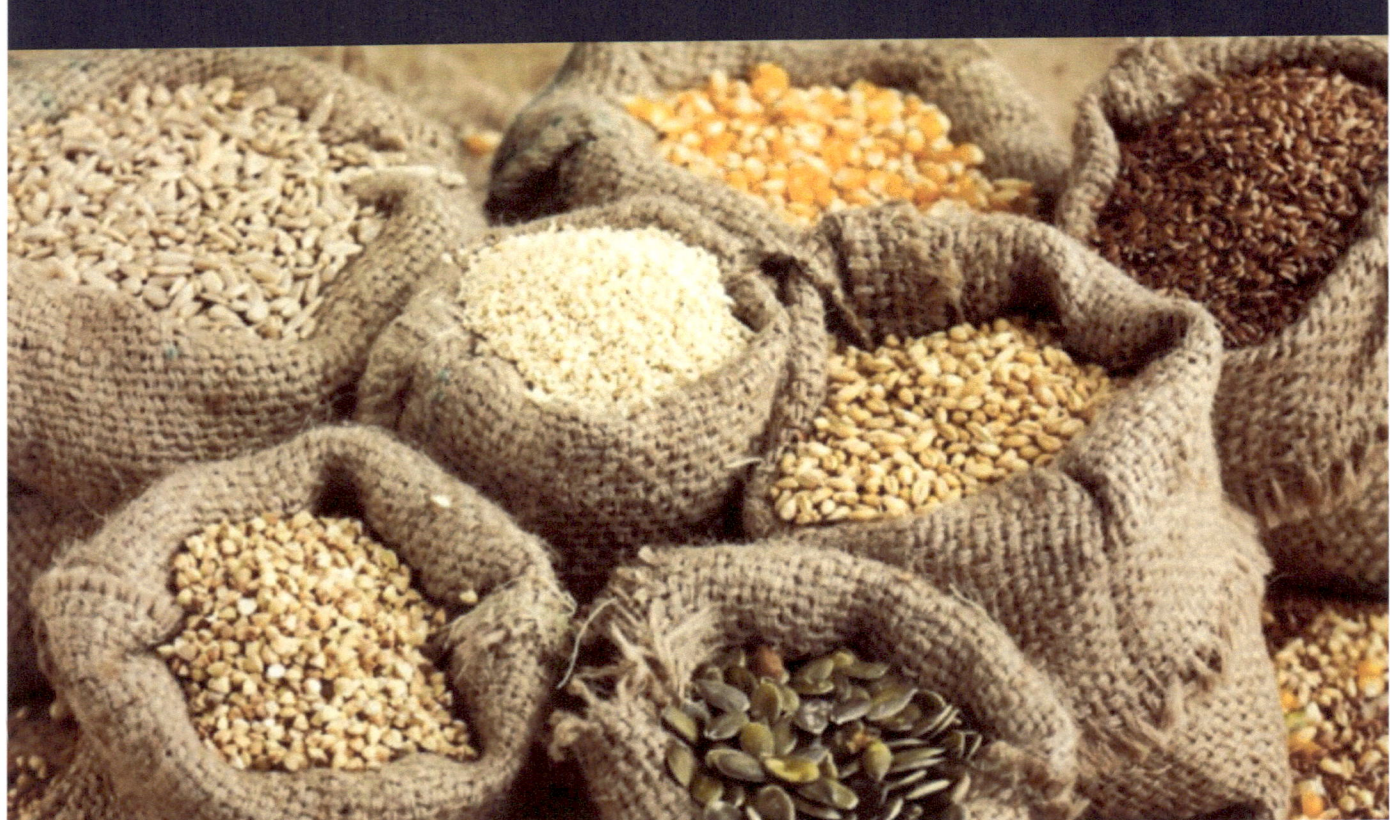

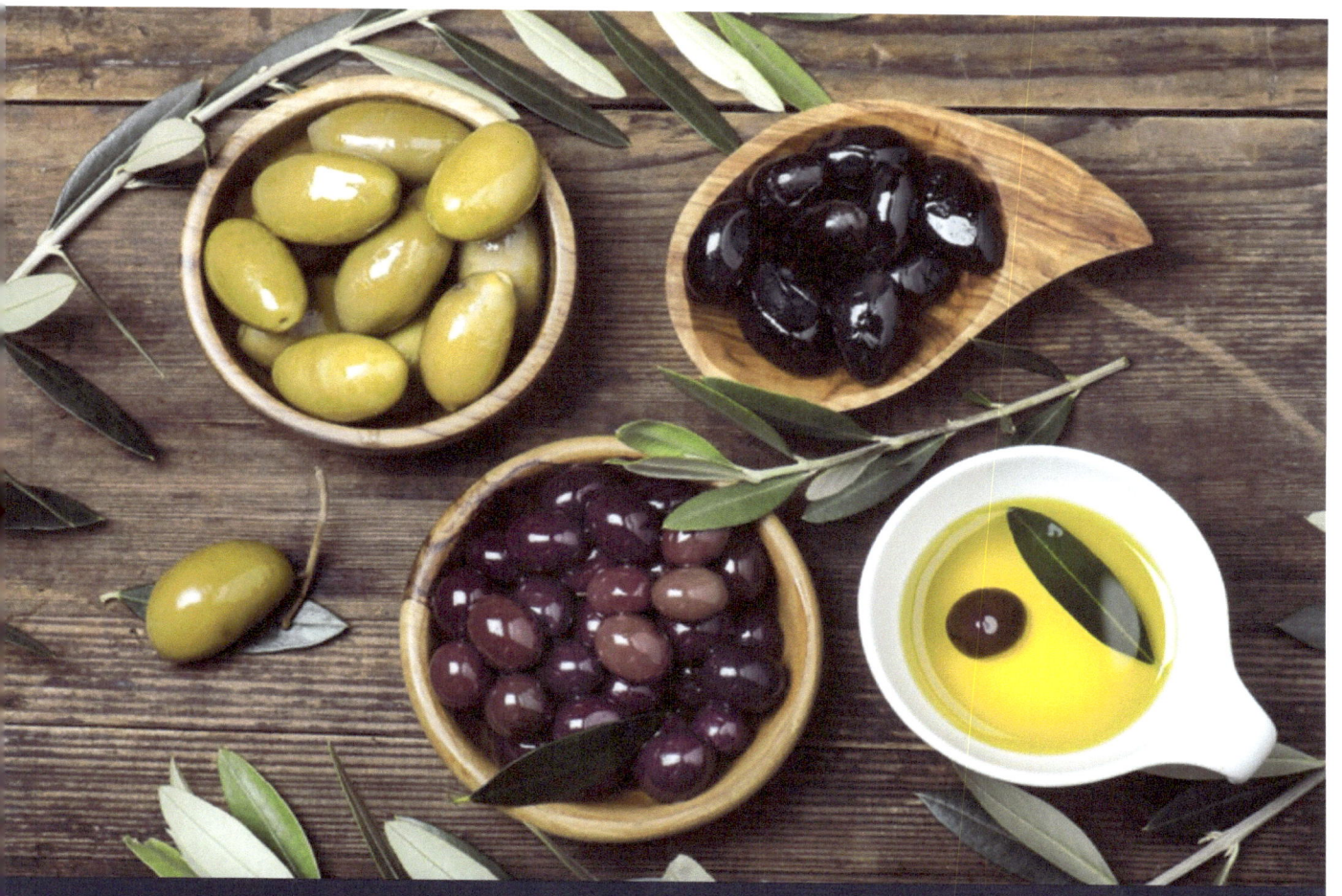

24
OLIVES AND OLIVE OIL

is a strong anti-inflammatory which its' compounds include at least nine different categories of polyphenols and more than twenty-four anti-inflammatory nutrients. It is also a good source of vitamin E which helps control uric acid levels and also provides a great amount of the anti-oxidant beta-carotenes.

www.ingramcontent.com/pod-product-compliance
Lightning Source LLC
Chambersburg PA
CBHW041319180526
45172CB00004B/1163